REAL FOOD FOR PREGNANCY

OPTIMAL NUTRITION FOR EVERY STAGE

MARY R. OWEN

TABLE OF CONTENT

INTRODUCTION

In the grand tapestry of life, few moments rival the profound transformation that occurs during pregnancy. It is a time of hope, of dreams, and of unparalleled connection between a mother and her unborn child. As nature orchestrates this wondrous symphony, it bestows upon women an extraordinary responsibility – the nurturing of a new life.

Real Food for Pregnancy is not just a book; it is a companion, a guide, and a celebration of the miraculous journey that is gestation. Within these pages, we embark on an exploration of nutrition, not as a regimen to be followed, but as an ode to the inherent wisdom of our bodies and the extraordinary potential they hold.

More than a mere collection of recipes, this book is a testament to the incredible power that real, whole foods possess. It is an invitation to rediscover the natural, unadulterated bounty that the earth provides, and to embrace it as the foundation of a healthy, thriving pregnancy.

Throughout these chapters, we will delve into the science that underpins the choices we make about what we eat. We will explore the nutrients that play pivotal roles in the development of your baby's body and brain, and in supporting your own vitality. From the essential vitamins and minerals to the crucial macronutrients, we will uncover the secrets of nourishment that have been passed down through generations.

But this book goes beyond scientific jargon and dietary charts. It speaks to the heart of motherhood, acknowledging the challenges and concerns that accompany this sacred time. It recognizes that, in addition to nourishing your growing child, you must also nurture your own well-being, your joy, and your sense of self.

Drawing on a wealth of research, expert interviews, and the collective wisdom of mothers around the world, Real Food for Pregnancy offers a holistic approach to nutrition. It takes into account the diverse needs and preferences of women from all walks of life and provides adaptable strategies to suit your unique circumstances.

As you embark on this transformative journey, remember that you are not alone. You are part of a vast, interconnected community of mothers, each weaving her own story into the rich tapestry of human experience. This book is here to guide you, to support you, and to celebrate you.

So, with an open heart and a hungry mind, let us begin this journey together. Let us embrace the power of real food to nourish not only the body, but also the spirit, as we embark on the most incredible adventure of our lives.

CHAPTER ONE

PREPARING FOR PREGNANCY

Preparing for pregnancy is a transformative journey that involves various facets of physical, emotional, and psychological well-being. Among these, nutrition plays a pivotal role in setting the stage for a healthy conception, pregnancy, and ultimately, the well-being of the developing fetus. This note aims to provide comprehensive guidance on the crucial aspect of optimal nutrition as the foundation for a successful and healthy pregnancy.

I. Preconception Nutrition:

Balanced Diet:

Prior to conception, it is imperative to adopt a well-balanced diet rich in essential nutrients like folic acid, iron, calcium, and omega-3 fatty acids. This provides the necessary foundation for the developing embryo.

Folic Acid Supplementation:

Folic acid is vital for preventing neural tube defects in the early stages of fetal development. Women of childbearing age should consider supplementation, ideally at least one month before conception.

Limiting Processed Foods and Sugars:

Reducing the intake of processed foods and sugars helps regulate blood sugar levels, which is crucial for reproductive health.

II. Essential Nutrients for Pregnancy:

Folate and Iron:

Folate aids in the formation of the neural tube and red blood cells, while iron prevents anaemia in both mother and baby. Green leafy vegetables, fortified cereals, and lean meats are excellent sources.

Calcium:

Vital for the development of the baby's bones and teeth, calcium can be found in dairy products, fortified plant-based milk, and leafy greens.

Omega-3 Fatty Acids:

These play a critical role in the development of the baby's brain and nervous system. Salmon and other fatty fish, chia seeds, and walnuts are good sources.

Protein:

Essential for tissue repair and growth, lean meats, poultry, fish, dairy, and plant-based sources like legumes and tofu should be included.

Vitamin D:

Supports bone health and immune function. Sun exposure, fortified dairy, and supplements if necessary, can ensure adequate levels.

III. Hydration and Fluid Intake:

Adequate Water Consumption:

Staying well-hydrated is crucial during pregnancy. Digestion, circulation, and the generation of amniotic fluid are all aided by water.

Limiting Caffeine and Alcohol:

High caffeine and alcohol intake can have adverse effects on fetal development. It is advised to limit or eliminate these during pregnancy.

IV. Managing Weight:

Maintaining a Healthy Weight:

Being either underweight or overweight can lead to complications during pregnancy. Achieving a healthy weight before conception reduces the risk of gestational diabetes, high blood pressure, and other complications.

Consulting a Healthcare Provider:

It is important to consult a healthcare provider for personalized advice regarding weight management and nutrition.

Optimal nutrition forms the bedrock of a healthy pregnancy. A well-balanced diet, coupled with appropriate supplements and lifestyle choices, lays the foundation for the well-being of both mother and baby. Remember, each pregnancy is unique, and consulting a healthcare provider is crucial for personalized guidance and support throughout this incredible journey. By prioritizing nutrition, you're not only preparing for a healthy pregnancy but also setting the stage for a bright and thriving future for your child.

PRECONCEPTION PLANNING

Preconception planning is an essential step towards ensuring a healthy and successful pregnancy. It involves making conscious choices and taking necessary steps before conceiving, with the aim of optimizing the health of both the prospective mother and father. This process lays the foundation for a safe and thriving pregnancy, reducing potential risks and complications. In this note, we will explore the significance of preconception planning, outlining key aspects, recommendations, and the benefits it brings to the overall reproductive journey.

Understanding Preconception Planning:

Preconception planning is a proactive approach to address various factors that can influence the health of the parents-to-be and the developing foetus. It typically begins several months before attempting to conceive. This period allows individuals or couples to make positive lifestyle changes, identify and manage potential health concerns, and establish a conducive environment for a healthy pregnancy.

Key Aspects of Preconception Planning:

Health Assessment and Screening:

Both partners should undergo a thorough health evaluation, including a review of medical history, physical examination, and any necessary tests or screenings.

Screening for pre-existing conditions such as diabetes, hypertension, and genetic disorders is crucial.

Nutrition and Diet:

A balanced, nutrient-rich diet is fundamental for preconception health. This includes a variety of fruits, vegetables, whole grains, lean proteins, and essential vitamins and minerals like folic acid, iron, and calcium.

Avoidance of harmful substances like excessive caffeine, alcohol, and tobacco is imperative.

Exercise and Physical Activity:

Regular physical activity promotes overall well-being and can contribute to a healthy pregnancy. It helps in maintaining a healthy weight, managing stress, and enhancing fertility.

Optimal Weight Management:

Achieving and maintaining a healthy weight is essential for fertility. Both being underweight and being overweight can mess with your hormones and impair your fertility.

Supplementation:

Folic acid and other essential vitamins and minerals should be included in the preconception plan to reduce the risk of neural tube defects and other developmental issues.

Immunizations and Vaccinations: Ensuring that both partners are up-to-date on vaccinations can prevent potential complications during pregnancy.

Mental and Emotional Well-being:

Stress management, relaxation techniques, and seeking emotional support are crucial components of preconception planning. A stable emotional state positively impacts fertility and sets the stage for a healthy pregnancy.

Environmental Factors:

Identifying and minimizing exposure to environmental toxins, pollutants, and chemicals is important. This includes avoiding hazardous workplaces and adopting safe household practices.

Benefits of Preconception Planning:

Reduced Pregnancy Complications:

Preconception planning significantly lowers the risk of complications such as gestational diabetes, preeclampsia, and preterm birth.

Healthy Foetal Development:

A well-prepared preconception phase provides an optimal environment for fetal growth and development.

Increased Fertility:

Addressing health concerns and making necessary lifestyle changes can enhance fertility, increasing the chances of successful conception.

Early Detection and Management of Risks:

Identifying and addressing any existing health conditions or potential risks before conception allows for timely intervention and management

Preconception planning is a vital step in the journey towards a healthy pregnancy. By focusing on various aspects of health and lifestyle, prospective parents can significantly increase their chances of a successful conception and ensure the best possible start for their future child. Consulting with healthcare professionals and seeking their guidance in this phase can provide valuable insights and personalized recommendations, ensuring a safe and joyful pregnancy experience.

THE ROLE OF MICRONUTRIENTS IN PRECONCEPTION HEALTH

Preconception health encompasses the period of time before a woman becomes pregnant. It is a critical phase that lays the foundation for a healthy pregnancy and the overall well-being of the developing foetus. Micronutrients, which include essential vitamins and minerals required in small quantities, play a pivotal role in ensuring optimal preconception health. In this note, we will explore the significance of various micronutrients and their impact on maternal and fetal health during this crucial period.

Folic Acid: A Cornerstone Micronutrient

One of the most well-known and widely studied micronutrients in preconception health is folic acid, a B-vitamin that is instrumental in preventing neural tube defects (NTDs) in developing fetuses. Adequate levels of folic acid in the mother's body prior to conception are essential, as NTDs often occur in the earliest stages of pregnancy when a woman may not even be aware she is pregnant. The recommended daily intake of folic acid for women planning to conceive is 400 micrograms, and it is commonly recommended to begin supplementation at least one month before conception.

Iron: Vital for Oxygen Transport and Cellular Function

Iron is an essential mineral crucial for the formation of haemoglobin, which carries oxygen to body tissues. The body requires much more iron during pregnancy to support the developing foetus and placenta. Preconception health should ideally ensure that a woman's iron stores are at an optimal level, as iron deficiency anemia can lead to complications like preterm birth and low birth weight. Including iron-rich foods in the diet and, if necessary, iron supplements can help maintain adequate iron levels.

Calcium and vitamin D: Creating Healthy Teeth and Strong Bones

Calcium and vitamin D are indispensable for the development of a healthy skeletal system in the foetus. Adequate calcium intake is crucial for the formation of bones and teeth, while vitamin D ensures proper absorption of calcium. Preconception health efforts should include a balanced intake of dairy products, leafy greens, and fortified foods, along with safe sun exposure, to ensure sufficient levels of these essential micronutrients.

Vitamin B12: Essential for Neurological Development

Vitamin B12 is vital for neurological development and is particularly important during the early stages of pregnancy. A deficiency in this vitamin can lead to serious neurological abnormalities in the developing foetus. Preconception health measures should aim to ensure that women, especially those following vegetarian or vegan diets, have adequate levels of vitamin B12. This can be achieved through dietary intake or supplementation.

Iodine: Critical for Thyroid Function and Cognitive Development

Iodine is essential for the production of thyroid hormones, which play a crucial role in fetal brain development. Severe iodine deficiency in pregnancy can lead to intellectual disabilities in the child. Ensuring adequate iodine intake before conception is therefore essential for preconception health. Iodized salt and seafood are common dietary sources of iodine.

Micronutrients form the cornerstone of preconception health, playing a pivotal role in the health and development of both the mother and the developing fetus. Folic acid, iron, calcium, vitamin D, vitamin B12, and iodine are among the key micronutrients that require special attention during this critical phase. It is imperative that women planning to conceive receive proper education and support to optimize their micronutrient status, thereby laying a strong foundation for a healthy pregnancy and ensuring the well-being of the future generation.

CHAPTER TWO

FIRST TRIMESTER: NOURISHING THE EARLY STAGE OF GROWTH

Early pregnancy is a critical period of rapid development and growth for the fetus. Proper nutrition during this phase is essential for ensuring the health and well-being of both the mother and the developing baby. This comprehensive guide aims to provide an in-depth overview of the nutritional needs during early pregnancy and offers practical tips to meet these requirements.

Folic Acid (Folate):

The early growth of the baby's neural tube, which eventually gives rise to the brain and spinal cord, depends on folic acid.

Recommended intake: 600-800 micrograms per day.

Sources: Leafy green vegetables, fortified cereals, beans, lentils, and citrus fruits.

It is advisable to start taking folic acid supplements before conception and continue during the first trimester.

Iron:

Haemoglobin, the substance that delivers oxygen to both the mother and the fetus, is made with the help of iron.

Recommended intake: 27 milligrams per day.

Sources: Lean meats, poultry, fish, beans, lentils, and fortified cereals.

Iron supplements may be prescribed if there's a deficiency, but consult a healthcare provider before starting any supplementation.

Calcium:

Calcium is vital for the development of the baby's bones and teeth.

Recommended intake: 1,000 milligrams per day.

Sources: Dairy products like milk, yogurt, cheese, leafy green vegetables, and fortified plant-based milk alternatives.

Protein:

Protein is essential for the growth of maternal and fetal tissues.

Recommended intake: About 75-100 grams per day, depending on the individual's weight and activity level.

Sources: Lean meats, poultry, fish, eggs, dairy products, legumes, nuts, and seeds.

Omega-3 Fatty Acids:

Omega-3 fatty acids, particularly DHA (docosahexaenoic acid), support brain and eye development in the foetus.

Sources: Fatty fish like salmon, mackerel, sardines, walnuts, chia seeds, and flaxseeds.

If dietary intake is insufficient, omega-3 supplements may be considered under medical guidance.

Vitamin D:

Vitamin D aids in the absorption of calcium and is crucial for bone health in both the mother and baby.

Recommended intake: 600-800 IU (International Units) per day.

Sources: Sun exposure, fortified dairy products, fatty fish, and vitamin D supplements if levels are low.

Vitamin C:

Vitamin C supports the absorption of iron from plant-based sources and helps in tissue repair.

Sources: Citrus fruits, strawberries, bell peppers, and tomatoes.

Vitamin A:

The growth of a baby's eyes, skin, and immune system depend on vitamin A

Sources: Sweet potatoes, carrots, spinach, and eggs. Avoid excessive intake of liver, as it can be high in vitamin A.

Fiber:

Adequate fiber intake helps prevent constipation and promotes healthy digestion.

Sources: Whole grains, fruits, vegetables, and legumes.

Hydration:

Staying well-hydrated is crucial for maintaining amniotic fluid levels, supporting blood volume expansion, and preventing dehydration.

Aim for at least 8-10 glasses of water per day, or more if required.

Meeting the nutritional needs during early pregnancy is fundamental for ensuring optimal maternal health and foetal development. A balanced diet rich in essential nutrients, along with appropriate supplementation if advised by a healthcare provider, plays a pivotal role in promoting a healthy pregnancy. It is always recommended to consult with a healthcare professional for personalized advice and guidance tailored to individual needs and circumstances.

MANAGING MORNING SICKNESS AND FOOD AVERSIONS

Managing morning sickness and food aversion in the first trimester of pregnancy is a common concern for many expectant mothers. This period can be challenging, as hormonal changes and increased sensitivity to certain smells and tastes can lead to nausea and vomiting. However, there are several strategies and tips to help alleviate these symptoms and ensure a more comfortable and healthy pregnancy.

1. Understand the Causes: Morning sickness, which can occur at any time of the day, is thought to be primarily caused by hormonal changes, particularly increased levels of human chorionic gonadotropin (hCG). Food aversions are often a natural response to protect the developing foetus from potential toxins. Understanding the underlying causes can help you cope better.

2. Small, Frequent Meals: Eating smaller, more frequent meals throughout the day can help regulate blood sugar levels and prevent the stomach from becoming too empty,

which can exacerbate nausea. Consider eating every 2-3 hours, even if it's just a small snack.

3. Ginger: Ginger is a natural remedy known for its anti-nausea properties. You can try ginger tea, ginger candies, or ginger supplements to help alleviate morning sickness. Many pregnant women find ginger to be quite effective.

4. Hydration: Staying hydrated is crucial during pregnancy. Sip water or clear fluids throughout the day to prevent dehydration, but avoid drinking large amounts of fluids at once, as this can trigger nausea. If plain water is unappealing, try flavoured water or electrolyte drinks.

5. Choose the Right Foods: Opt for bland, easily digestible foods like crackers, plain toast, rice, or applesauce. Avoid spicy, greasy, or highly aromatic foods that may trigger nausea. Eating cold or room temperature foods can also be less nauseating than hot dishes.

6. Protein-Rich Snacks: Protein can help stabilize blood sugar levels and reduce

nausea. Consider snacks like yogurt, nuts, or lean meats to keep your energy levels up and manage morning sickness.

7. Acupressure Bands: Some women find relief from morning sickness by wearing acupressure bands on their wrists. These bands apply gentle pressure to specific points that may help alleviate nausea.

8. Aromatherapy: Certain scents can either alleviate or exacerbate morning sickness. Experiment with different scents, such as lemon, peppermint, or lavender, to see if any of them help you feel better.

9. Rest and Stress Reduction: Getting enough rest is crucial during pregnancy. Fatigue can exacerbate nausea, so make sure you're getting adequate sleep. Managing stress through relaxation techniques like deep breathing, yoga, or meditation can also help reduce symptoms.

10. Consult Your Healthcare Provider: If your morning sickness is severe and persistent, consult your healthcare provider.

They can offer guidance and may prescribe anti-nausea medications that are safe for pregnancy.

11. Supplement with Prenatal Vitamins: Taking prenatal vitamins as recommended by your healthcare provider can ensure you're getting the necessary nutrients, even when your diet is limited due to food aversions.

12. Support System: Don't hesitate to seek support from your partner, family, and friends. They can assist with meal preparation and household chores during this challenging time.

13. Keep Track: Maintain a diary to identify any specific triggers for your morning sickness and food aversions. This can help you avoid those triggers and make better dietary choices.

14. Be Patient: Remember that morning sickness is a temporary phase in pregnancy for most women. It typically improves after the first trimester. Be patient with yourself and do what you can to manage the symptoms.

In conclusion, managing morning sickness and food aversion in the first trimester of pregnancy can be challenging, but with the right strategies and support, you can navigate this phase more comfortably. Always consult your healthcare provider for personalized advice and to rule out any underlying medical issues. This period is just one step on the journey to motherhood, and it's important to prioritize your health and well-being.

BUILDING A STRONG FOUNDATION FOR FOETAL DEVELOPMENT

The first trimester of pregnancy is a critical period for the development of the fetus. During this time, the foundation for the baby's growth and well-being is laid. It is essential for expectant mothers to adopt a proactive and holistic approach to ensure optimal foetal development. This note will outline key considerations and practices that play a pivotal role in establishing a strong foundation for foetal development during the first trimester.

Prenatal Care: Early and regular prenatal care is paramount for both the mother's health and the optimal development of the foetus. This includes scheduled visits to healthcare providers, comprehensive health assessments, and guidance on healthy lifestyle choices.

Proper Nutrition: A balanced and nutritious diet is crucial in the first trimester. It is recommended to increase intake of folic acid, iron, calcium, and other essential nutrients. Foods rich in folate, such as leafy greens and legumes, are vital for neural tube development. Adequate protein, healthy fats, and a variety of fruits and vegetables contribute to overall growth and development.

Folic Acid Supplementation: Folic acid is a B-vitamin that aids in preventing neural tube defects. Taking the recommended dosage (typically 400-800 micrograms) before and during early pregnancy is vital. If not obtained through diet alone, supplements should be taken under the guidance of a healthcare provider.

Avoiding Harmful Substances: The first trimester is a critical period of organogenesis, and exposure to harmful substances can have detrimental effects. Smoking, alcohol consumption, illicit drugs, and certain prescription medications can pose significant risks to fetal development. It is imperative for expectant mothers to abstain from these substances.

Managing Stress: High levels of stress can impact fetal development. Engaging in relaxation techniques such as deep breathing exercises, meditation, and prenatal yoga can help reduce stress levels. Adequate rest and sleep are equally important in maintaining a healthy pregnancy.

Exercise and Physical Activity: Regular, moderate-intensity exercise is generally safe and beneficial during pregnancy. Activities like walking, swimming, and prenatal yoga can improve cardiovascular health, boost mood, and promote overall well-being.

However, it is essential to consult a healthcare provider for personalized advice.

Avoiding Environmental Hazards: Pregnant women should be cautious about exposure to environmental toxins, such as pesticides, solvents, and radiation. Minimizing contact with these substances, particularly in the workplace, is crucial for foetal development.

Genetic Screening and Counseling: Early prenatal genetic screening can identify potential risks and conditions that may affect the baby's development. Genetic counseling can provide valuable information and guidance for families facing specific genetic concerns.

Monitoring Medical Conditions: Expectant mothers with pre-existing medical conditions, such as diabetes or hypertension, require specialized care and monitoring. Proper management of these conditions is essential for a healthy pregnancy and optimal fetal development.

The first trimester of pregnancy lays the foundation for a healthy and thriving baby. Through early and regular prenatal care, a balanced diet, and the avoidance of harmful substances, expectant mothers can significantly impact their baby's development. By adopting a holistic approach to pregnancy, women can ensure the best possible start for their child's lifelong journey of growth and well-being. Consulting with healthcare professionals and following their guidance is crucial in navigating this transformative period.

CHAPTER THREE

SECOND TRIMESTER: SUPPORTING GROWTH AND VITALITY

The second trimester of pregnancy, spanning from weeks 13 to 27, is a critical period marked by significant physiological and anatomical changes in both the mother and the developing fetus. During this time, the demands on maternal and fetal growth undergo a dynamic transformation to accommodate the rapidly evolving needs of both entities.

Maternal Physiological Changes

Cardiovascular System: One of the most notable changes during the second trimester is the increased cardiac output. This is primarily driven by an expansion in blood volume to meet the demands of the growing fetus. The heart experiences an elevated stroke volume and heart rate, resulting in a higher cardiac output. This physiological adaptation is crucial for ensuring an adequate supply of oxygen and nutrients to the developing fetus.

Respiratory System: The growing uterus begins to exert pressure on the diaphragm, leading to a feeling of breathlessness in some pregnant individuals. However, the maternal respiratory rate does not significantly increase, suggesting that adaptations in tidal volume compensate for the reduced diaphragmatic excursion.

Endocrine System: The second trimester is characterized by a surge in placental hormone production, particularly human chorionic gonadotropin (hCG), estrogen, and progesterone. These hormones play crucial roles in maintaining pregnancy, promoting fetal development, and preparing the body for labor and lactation.

Metabolic Changes: Maternal metabolism undergoes notable alterations to support the growing fetus. Insulin sensitivity decreases, leading to a physiological state termed "insulin resistance". This allows for a greater availability of glucose for fetal growth. Additionally, there is an increase in maternal fat stores, which serve as an energy reserve during the later stages of pregnancy.

Fetal Growth and Development

Organogenesis Completion: By the end of the first trimester, the majority of the fetal organs have formed, and during the second trimester, they undergo significant growth and differentiation. This includes the development of specialized tissues and the initiation of physiological functions.

Rapid Growth Phase: The second trimester is often referred to as the "honeymoon period" of pregnancy due to the reduction in common first-trimester discomforts. During this time, the fetus experiences a remarkable growth spurt, with a significant increase in weight, length, and overall body mass.

Central Nervous System Maturation: The fetal brain experiences a phase of rapid growth and maturation during the second trimester. Neuronal connections multiply, and structures such as the cerebral cortex develop more defined layers. This period is critical for cognitive and neurological development.

Vernix Caseosa and Lanugo Formation: Around the 20th week, the fetus begins to produce vernix caseosa, a protective waxy substance that covers the skin. Additionally, fine hair known as lanugo appears to aid in temperature regulation.

Nutritional Demands and Considerations

Increased Caloric Intake: The second trimester sees a rise in the energy requirements for both the mother and fetus. An additional 300-500 calories per day are recommended to support fetal growth and maternal metabolic needs.

Nutrient-Dense Diet: Adequate intake of essential nutrients such as folic acid, iron, calcium, and omega-3 fatty acids is crucial for the development of the fetus and the maintenance of maternal health.

Hydration: Proper hydration is essential to support the increased blood volume and amniotic fluid production, as well as to aid in the transport of nutrients to the fetus.

In summary, the second trimester of pregnancy represents a period of rapid growth and development for both the mother and the fetus. Physiological adaptations in the maternal cardiovascular, respiratory, and endocrine systems, as well as fetal organ maturation, highlight the intricate interplay between the two entities. Adequate nutrition and prenatal care are paramount to ensuring a healthy pregnancy outcome during this critical phase.

ADDRESSING COMMON DISCOMFORTS AND CHALLENGES

The second trimester of pregnancy is often referred to as the "golden period" due to the reduction of early pregnancy symptoms and the onset of a newfound sense of well-being. However, this phase is not without its own set of challenges and discomforts. This note aims to provide comprehensive guidance on addressing and managing these issues, ensuring a smoother pregnancy experience for expectant mothers.

Morning Sickness and Nausea:

While morning sickness typically subsides in the second trimester, some may still experience mild nausea. Staying hydrated and eating small, frequent meals can be beneficial.

Ginger, lemon, and mint can be natural remedies to alleviate nausea. Any herbal therapies should be used after consulting a healthcare professional.

Fatigue and Low Energy:

Adequate rest and sleep are crucial during this phase. Taking short naps and practicing relaxation techniques can help combat fatigue.

Engaging in light exercise, such as prenatal yoga or swimming, can boost energy levels.

Backaches and Body Pain:

As the uterus expands, it puts strain on the back. Practicing good posture and using a supportive chair and pillows can alleviate back pain.

Gentle exercises to strengthen the core and back muscles, as well as prenatal massages, can provide relief.

Leg Cramps and Swelling:

Staying hydrated, maintaining a balanced diet, and regular exercise can help reduce leg cramps and swelling.

Elevating the legs, avoiding prolonged standing or sitting, and wearing comfortable shoes can prevent or alleviate discomfort.

Mood Swings and Emotional Changes:

Hormonal fluctuations can lead to mood swings. Engaging in activities that bring joy, seeking support from loved ones, and practicing mindfulness can help stabilize emotions.

Open communication with a partner or healthcare provider about emotional well-being is crucial.

Skin Changes and Stretch Marks:

Regularly moisturizing the skin, especially areas prone to stretching, can help prevent stretch marks. Using creams rich in vitamin E and cocoa butter can be beneficial.

Staying hydrated and maintaining a balanced diet can promote healthy skin.

Heartburn and Indigestion:

Eating smaller, more frequent meals and avoiding spicy or greasy foods can help alleviate heartburn.

Sitting upright after meals and avoiding tight clothing around the waist can also provide relief.

Increased Libido and Sexual Discomfort:

Many women experience an increase in libido during the second trimester. Open communication with a partner and exploring comfortable positions can maintain intimacy.

If there is discomfort or concerns, consulting a healthcare provider is essential.

Gestational Diabetes and Blood Pressure:

Regular prenatal check-ups are crucial for monitoring blood pressure and blood sugar levels.

Following a balanced diet, staying active, and managing stress can help regulate blood sugar and blood pressure.

The second trimester of pregnancy brings its own set of challenges, but with proper care and attention, many of these discomforts can be managed effectively. It is essential for expectant mothers to listen to their bodies, seek support, and consult their healthcare providers for personalized advice. By addressing these common issues, women can navigate this phase with confidence, ensuring a healthy and enjoyable pregnancy experience.

BALANCING MACRO AND MICRONUTRIENTS FOR OPTIMAL HEALTH

Pregnancy is a transformative period in a woman's life, marked by numerous physiological changes and increased nutritional demands. The significance of a balanced diet during this time cannot be overstated. It not only supports the mother's health but also plays a pivotal role in the development of the foetus. Achieving the right balance of macro and micronutrients is crucial for both maternal and foetal well-being.

Macros: The Foundation of a Healthy Pregnancy

Carbohydrates

Carbohydrates are the body's primary source of energy. During pregnancy, they become even more essential as they provide the necessary fuel for both the mother and the growing foetus. Choosing complex carbohydrates over simple ones is a good idea. These sources release energy slowly, helping stabilize blood sugar levels and preventing sudden spikes or crashes.

Proteins

Proteins are the building blocks of life. They are crucial for the development of the fetus's organs, tissues, and overall growth. Additionally, proteins support the mother's own tissue expansion and blood volume increase. Include lean meats, poultry, fish, legumes, and dairy products in your diet to ensure an adequate supply of essential amino acids.

Fats

Healthy fats are vital for brain development in the fetus and the absorption of fat-soluble vitamins. Walnuts, flaxseeds, and fatty fish are good sources of omega-3 fatty acids. Saturated and trans fats should be limited, as they can contribute to gestational complications.

Micronutrients: The Mighty Essentials

Folate (Vitamin B9)

Early in a pregnancy, folate is essential for the formation of the neural tube. Inadequate folate intake can lead to neural tube defects. Leafy greens, legumes, fortified cereals, and supplements prescribed by healthcare professionals can help meet the increased folate requirements during pregnancy.

Iron

The demand for iron rises significantly during pregnancy due to increased blood volume and the needs of the developing foetus. A deficiency can lead to anaemia, which can have serious consequences for both mother and baby. Red meat, poultry, fish, beans, and iron-fortified cereals are excellent sources of iron.

Calcium

Calcium is essential for the development of the baby's bones, teeth, and muscles. If the mother's calcium intake is inadequate, the baby will draw from the mother's own calcium stores, potentially leading to health issues for the mother. Dairy products, leafy greens, fortified plant-based milk, and calcium supplements can help meet the recommended daily intake.

Vitamins (especially A, C, D, and E)

These vitamins play various critical roles in pregnancy:

Vitamin A supports foetal vision, immune function, and tissue repair. However, excessive intake can be harmful, so it's important to get it from food sources like sweet potatoes, carrots, and leafy greens.

Vitamin C aids in collagen formation, absorption of iron, and supports the immune system. Excellent sources include strawberries, bell peppers, and citrus fruits.

The immune system, healthy bones, and calcium absorption all depend on vitamin D. Sun exposure and fortified dairy or plant-based milk can provide the necessary vitamin D.

Antioxidant vitamin E aids in preventing cell deterioration. Nuts, seeds, and spinach are good sources.

Hydration: The Unsung Hero

Adequate hydration is often overlooked but is crucial during pregnancy. It supports the increased blood volume, amniotic fluid, and the body's cooling mechanisms. Water, herbal teas, and hydrating fruits and vegetables are excellent choices.

Consultation with Healthcare Professionals

It's imperative to consult with healthcare providers to tailor nutritional recommendations to individual needs. Factors like pre-existing health conditions, multiple pregnancies, and dietary restrictions can influence specific nutrient requirements.

In conclusion, achieving optimal health during pregnancy hinges on a well-balanced diet rich in both macro and micronutrients. A mindful and diverse selection of whole foods, complemented by appropriate supplements when necessary, ensures a smooth and healthy pregnancy journey. Remember, the best foundation for a thriving baby is a nourished and healthy mother.

CHAPTER FOUR

THIRD TRIMESTER: PREPARING FOR BIRTH AND BEYOND

Late pregnancy, also known as the third trimester, is a crucial period in a woman's gestational journey. During this time, the developing fetus experiences rapid growth and development, placing increased demands on the mother's body for essential nutrients. Meeting these escalating nutritional needs is paramount for the health and well-being of both the mother and the developing baby. This note aims to provide a comprehensive overview of the key nutrients required during late pregnancy and strategies to ensure their adequate intake.

Caloric Intake:

The caloric needs of a pregnant woman increase in the third trimester to support the growing fetus and the changes in the mother's body.

A balanced diet that includes a variety of nutrient-dense foods is essential to meet these increased energy demands.

Protein:

Adequate protein intake is crucial for fetal growth, especially in the late stages of pregnancy when the rate of growth is most rapid.

Sources of high-quality protein include lean meats, fish, eggs, dairy products, legumes, and plant-based protein alternatives.

Calcium:

Calcium is vital for the development of the baby's bones and teeth, as well as for maintaining the mother's own bone health.

Dairy products, leafy greens, fortified cereals, and nuts are excellent sources of calcium.

Iron:

Iron requirements increase significantly in late pregnancy to support the expansion of the mother's blood volume and to ensure adequate oxygen supply to the fetus.

Foods rich in heme iron (found in animal products) and non-heme iron (found in plant-based foods) should be included in the diet. Iron-fortified cereals and legumes are also valuable sources.

Folate and Folic Acid:

Adequate folate intake is crucial in preventing neural tube defects in the developing foetus.

Foods rich in folate include dark leafy greens, legumes, citrus fruits, and fortified cereals. Folic acid supplements may also be recommended by healthcare providers.

Omega-3 Fatty Acids:

DHA (docosahexaenoic acid), in particular, is an omega-3 fatty acid that is crucial for the growth of the baby's brain and eyes.

Omega-3 fatty acids are abundant in fatty fish like salmon, mackerel, and sardines as well as flaxseeds and walnuts.

Vitamin D:

Vitamin D is crucial for calcium absorption, which is essential for the development of the baby's bones and teeth.

Sun exposure and dietary sources like fatty fish, fortified dairy products, and supplements are important for maintaining adequate vitamin D levels.

Vitamin C:

Vitamin C aids in the absorption of nonheme iron, making it an important nutrient for preventing iron deficiency anemia.

Excellent sources of vitamin C are broccoli, bell peppers, strawberries, citrus fruits, and strawberries.

Fluid Intake:

Staying well-hydrated is crucial for the mother's overall health and for maintaining the amniotic fluid levels that protect the developing baby.

Supplementation:

Prenatal supplements are often recommended during late pregnancy to ensure that all nutrient needs are met. These supplements should complement a balanced diet, not replace it.

Meeting the escalating nutritional needs in late pregnancy is of paramount importance for the health and well-being of both the mother and the developing baby. A balanced diet, rich in essential nutrients, combined with appropriate supplementation when necessary, forms the cornerstone of a healthy pregnancy. Consulting a healthcare provider for personalized advice and regular prenatal check-ups is essential in ensuring a smooth and healthy pregnancy journey.

MANAGING WEIGHT GAIN AND BLOOD SUGAR LEVEL

Managing weight and blood sugar levels during late pregnancy is crucial for the health of both the mother and the developing foetus. It requires a combination of a balanced diet, regular exercise, monitoring blood sugar levels, and appropriate medical supervision. Here's a comprehensive guide on how to effectively manage weight and blood sugar levels during late pregnancy:

Balanced Diet:

Focus on nutrient-dense, entire foods including fruits, vegetables, whole grains, lean meats, and healthy fats. These provide essential vitamins and minerals necessary for both you and your baby's development.

Fiber Intake: High-fiber foods help regulate blood sugar levels by slowing down digestion. Opt for whole grains, legumes, fruits, and vegetables.

Lean protein sources, such as poultry, fish, beans, and tofu, should be included in your diet. Protein helps maintain muscle mass and supports the growth of the fetus.

Limit Processed Foods: Minimize consumption of processed and sugary foods, as they can lead to rapid spikes and drops in blood sugar levels.

Regular Exercise:

Consult with a Healthcare Provider: Before starting any exercise routine, consult with your healthcare provider to ensure it is safe and appropriate for your individual circumstances.

Low-Impact Activities: Engage in low-impact exercises like walking, swimming, and prenatal yoga. These activities help regulate blood sugar levels and control weight gain.

Strength Training: Incorporate light strength training to maintain muscle mass and improve insulin sensitivity.

Blood Sugar Monitoring:

Frequent Testing: Regularly monitor your blood sugar levels as recommended by your healthcare provider. This might involve daily glucose checks, especially after meals.

Keep a Log: Maintain a record of your blood sugar levels, along with details of your meals, exercise routines, and any unusual symptoms. This information can be useful for both you and your healthcare provider in making adjustments to your care plan.

Gestational Diabetes Management:

Follow Medical Advice: If you have been diagnosed with gestational diabetes, follow your healthcare provider's recommendations regarding diet, exercise, and medication (if prescribed).

Nutritional Counseling: Work with a registered dietitian who specializes in gestational diabetes to create a personalized meal plan that helps stabilize blood sugar levels.

Hydration:

Adequate Water Intake: Staying properly hydrated is crucial during pregnancy. Water helps transport nutrients, regulate body temperature, and maintain amniotic fluid levels.

Stress Management:

Relaxation Techniques: Engage in relaxation techniques such as deep breathing exercises, prenatal massage, or meditation. High stress levels can impact blood sugar levels, so finding ways to relax is essential.

Medical Supervision:

Regular Prenatal Check-ups: Attend all scheduled prenatal check-ups and keep your healthcare provider informed of any changes or concerns.

Medication Management: If prescribed, take any medications as directed by your healthcare provider. This may include insulin injections or oral medications to manage blood sugar levels.

Rest and Sleep:

Adequate Sleep: Make sure you receive enough sleep. Fatigue and inadequate sleep can affect both blood sugar levels and overall well-being.

Consult a Registered Dietitian:

Individualized Guidance: A registered dietitian with expertise in pregnancy and gestational diabetes can provide personalized guidance on meal planning and blood sugar control.

Always keep in mind that every pregnancy is different and that what works for one person may not work for another. It's crucial to work closely with your healthcare provider to develop a plan tailored to your specific needs and circumstances. Following these guidelines can help promote a healthy pregnancy while effectively managing weight and blood sugar levels.

PREPARING FOR LABOUR, DELIVERY AND POSTPARTUM RECOVERY

The remarkable act of childbirth marks the culmination of the pregnant experience. To ensure a smooth transition into parenthood, it is crucial to be well-prepared for labour, delivery, and the postpartum period. This comprehensive guide aims to provide you with essential information and practical tips to help you navigate through this transformative experience.

I. Preparing for Labour:

Prenatal Education: Enrol in prenatal classes to learn about the stages of labour, pain management techniques, breathing exercises, and infant care basics.

Familiarize yourself with the signs of labour and when to contact your healthcare provider.

Create a Birth Plan: Outline your preferences for labour and delivery, including pain management options, birthing positions, and any special requests.

Discuss this plan with your healthcare provider and birthing team.

Physical and Mental Health: Maintain a balanced diet rich in nutrients essential for both you and your baby's health.

Engage in regular prenatal exercises, including yoga, swimming, and walking, to promote strength and flexibility.

Practice relaxation techniques such as deep breathing, meditation, or prenatal massage to reduce stress and anxiety.

Pack a Hospital Bag: Include essentials like comfortable clothing, toiletries, snacks, important documents, and items for the baby (e.g., clothes, diapers).

Arrange Transportation and Support:

Ensure you have a reliable mode of transportation to the hospital or birthing center.

Have a designated support person who will accompany you during labour.

II. Labour and Delivery:

Early Labour: Keep hydrated, have small snacks, and get as much shut-eye as you can.

Any modifications to your condition should be communicated to your healthcare professional.

Active Labour:

Utilize breathing techniques and position changes to manage pain.

Follow your birth plan, but remain flexible if circumstances require adjustments.

Pain Management Options:

Discuss pain relief choices with your healthcare provider, which may include natural techniques like hydrotherapy or medical options like epidurals.

Emotional Support: Lean on your support person, whether a partner, family member, or doula, for encouragement and comfort.

Postpartum Care Team: Familiarize yourself with the healthcare professionals who will be assisting during the birth, including doctors, nurses, and midwives.

III. Postpartum Recovery:

Immediate Postpartum Period: Rest and allow your body time to recover from the physical demands of labour.

Begin breastfeeding, if desired, with the help of a lactation consultant.

Pain Management and Healing: For pain relief, take prescribed drugs as instructed.

Practice gentle postpartum exercises to aid in recovery, under the guidance of your healthcare provider.

Emotional Well-being: Be mindful of the "baby blues" and postpartum depression. Seek professional support if needed.

Newborn Care and Parenting:

Learn about newborn care, including feeding, diapering, and sleeping routines.

Communicate openly with your partner about shared responsibilities and expectations.

Self-care and Support: Prioritize self-care activities like gentle exercises, nutritious meals, and adequate rest.

Connect with support groups, friends, and family members for emotional support and guidance.

Preparation is the cornerstone of a positive birthing experience and postpartum recovery. By equipping yourself with knowledge, seeking emotional and physical support, and remaining flexible in your approach, you can navigate this transformative journey with confidence and grace. Remember, every pregnancy and birth is unique, so trust your instincts and lean on your support network for guidance. Congratulations on this significant turning point in your life!

CHAPTER FIVE

A CLOSER LOOK AT NUTRITIONAL COMPONENT

MACRONUTRIENTS: PROTEINS

Pregnancy is a remarkable journey marked by significant physiological changes within a woman's body. One of the most fundamental aspects of a healthy pregnancy is proper nutrition. Among the various nutrients required, proteins play an especially crucial role. They serve as the building blocks for cells, tissues, and organs, supporting the growth and development of both the mother and the fetus. This note will delve into the impact of proteins on pregnancy, highlighting their essential functions and emphasizing their significance in ensuring a healthy and successful gestation period.

Protein's Role in Cell Growth and Repair

Proteins are composed of amino acids, which are essential for cell growth and repair. During pregnancy, the mother's body undergoes rapid cell division to accommodate the growing fetus. This process requires a substantial supply of amino acids, which can only be obtained through a protein-rich diet.

Formation of Foetal Tissues

The foetus undergoes a remarkable transformation throughout pregnancy, transitioning from a single fertilized cell to a complex organism. Proteins are indispensable for the formation of various foetal tissues, including muscles, bones, skin, and internal organs. Insufficient protein intake can hinder this crucial process, potentially leading to developmental issues.

Development of the Placenta

The placenta, a temporary organ that forms during pregnancy, plays a vital role in facilitating nutrient exchange between the mother and the foetus. Proteins are essential in the construction and maintenance of this crucial structure. A deficiency in protein intake may lead to inadequate placental development, potentially causing complications in fetal growth.

Hormone Regulation

Hormones such as insulin, growth hormone, and various enzymes are proteins or derived from proteins. These play a pivotal role in regulating metabolic processes, ensuring that both the mother and the foetus receive the necessary nutrients. Proper hormonal balance is crucial for a healthy pregnancy.

Blood Volume and Haemoglobin Synthesis

Pregnancy necessitates an expansion of blood volume to accommodate the increased nutrient and oxygen requirements of the foetus. Proteins are essential for the synthesis of haemoglobin, the protein responsible for carrying oxygen in the blood. Inadequate protein intake can lead to anaemia, which can have severe consequences for both the mother and the developing foetus.

Immune System Function

Pregnancy is a time when a woman's immune system undergoes significant changes to protect the fetus from potential threats. Proteins play a vital role in the production of antibodies, which help defend against infections and diseases. A protein-deficient diet can weaken the immune system, potentially putting both the mother and the foetus at risk.

Gestational Weight Gain and Maternal Health

Adequate protein intake is essential for achieving healthy gestational weight gain. It supports the growth of maternal tissues, including the uterus and breasts, which are vital for a successful pregnancy and lactation. Additionally, protein-rich foods can help stabilize blood sugar levels, reducing the risk of gestational diabetes

In summary, proteins are the cornerstone of a healthy pregnancy. Their multifaceted role in cell growth, tissue formation, hormonal regulation, and immune function underscores their critical importance. A balanced and protein-rich diet is essential to ensure the well-being and optimal development of both the mother and the foetus. It is imperative that pregnant women, in consultation with healthcare providers, pay careful attention to their protein intake, thereby laying a strong foundation for a healthy, successful pregnancy.

CARBOHYDRATE

Carbohydrates are one of the three essential macronutrients, alongside proteins and fats, that provide the body with energy. During pregnancy, the importance of a balanced diet cannot be overstated, and carbohydrates play a crucial role in ensuring the health and well-being of both the mother and the developing foetus.

Types of Carbohydrates:

Carbohydrates are classified into three main groups: sugars, starches, and dietary fiber. Sugars can be found in fruits, vegetables, and dairy products, as well as in processed foods as added sugars. Complex carbohydrates called starches are present in grains, legumes, and tubers. Dietary fiber, a non-digestible form of carbohydrate, is abundant in fruits, vegetables, and whole grains.

Role of Carbohydrates in Pregnancy:

Energy Source: Carbohydrates are the body's primary source of energy. During pregnancy, the demand for energy increases significantly to support the growth and development of the fetus. Complex carbohydrates provide a sustained release of energy, which helps maintain stable blood glucose levels.

Nutrient Absorption: Carbohydrates aid in the absorption of essential nutrients. They enhance the absorption of vital vitamins and minerals, such as B-complex vitamins, calcium, and iron, which are crucial for the development of the fetus and the overall health of the mother.

Preventing Ketosis: Inadequate carbohydrate intake may lead to the production of ketones, which can be harmful to both the mother and the foetus. Ketosis can result in a decrease in fetal growth and development, making it imperative for pregnant women to consume an adequate amount of carbohydrates.

Gestational Diabetes Management: A well-balanced intake of carbohydrates is essential for managing gestational diabetes. Monitoring the type and quantity of carbohydrates consumed can help regulate blood sugar levels, reducing the risk of complications for both mother and child.

Digestive Health: Dietary fiber, a type of carbohydrate, is crucial for maintaining healthy digestion. It prevents constipation, a common issue during pregnancy, and supports overall gastrointestinal health.

Reduction of Nausea and Vomiting: Complex carbohydrates, particularly those with a low glycemic index, can help alleviate morning sickness, a common symptom in early pregnancy.

Choosing the Right Carbohydrates:

Choose complex carbohydrates like whole grains, legumes, and starchy vegetables over simple carbohydrates. These deliver energy gradually, aiding in the stabilization of blood sugar levels.

Foods High in Fiber: Make sure your diet is full of fruits, vegetables, and whole grains.

These not only provide essential nutrients but also promote digestive health.

Limit Added Sugars: Minimize the consumption of foods and beverages with added sugars. These provide empty calories without the accompanying nutrients required during pregnancy.

Balanced Intake: Aim for a balanced intake of carbohydrates, proteins, and fats to ensure optimal nutrition for both the mother and the developing foetus.

Carbohydrates form a cornerstone of a healthy diet during pregnancy. They provide the energy needed for the increased metabolic demands of pregnancy and support the growth and development of the foetus. By making informed choices about the types and sources of carbohydrates consumed, expectant mothers can help ensure a healthy and successful pregnancy. Always consult a healthcare professional for personalized dietary recommendations during pregnancy.

Fats as a Macronutrient

Pregnancy is a critical period in a woman's life, characterized by increased nutritional needs to support both maternal health and fetal development. While it is crucial to focus on various aspects of nutrition during pregnancy, including proteins, carbohydrates, vitamins, and minerals, the role of fats as a macronutrient should not be underestimated.

Understanding Fats:

Fats, also known as lipids, are an essential macronutrient that serves several vital functions in the body. They are composed of fatty acids, which can be categorized into saturated, monounsaturated, and polyunsaturated fats. Each type of fatty acid plays a unique role in maintaining health.

II. The Importance of Fats During Pregnancy:

Energy Source:

Fats serve as a concentrated source of energy, providing more than twice the amount of energy per gram compared to carbohydrates or proteins. This is particularly important during pregnancy when a woman's energy needs are increased.

Foetal Brain and Nervous System Development:

Polyunsaturated fats, specifically omega-3 fatty acids like docosahexaenoic acid (DHA), are crucial for the development of the fetal brain and nervous system. These fats contribute significantly to cognitive development and visual acuity.

Cell Membrane Integrity:

Cell membrane function and structure both depend on fats. They help regulate what enters and exits cells, influencing nutrient transport and cellular communication, which is especially vital during the rapid cell division and growth occurring in foetal development.

Vitamin Absorption:

Certain fat-soluble vitamins, such as vitamins A, D, E, and K, require dietary fats for absorption. These vitamins play critical roles in immune function, bone health, vision, and blood clotting, all of which are crucial during pregnancy.

Hormone Production:

Fats are essential precursors for the production of various hormones, including those involved in regulating reproductive processes. Adequate fat intake is crucial for hormone balance during pregnancy.

Protection of Vital Organs:

The layer of fat around vital organs, known as visceral fat, provides cushioning and protection. This is especially important during pregnancy to safeguard both the mother and the developing foetus.

III. Types of Fats and Pregnancy:

Saturated Fats:

While saturated fats should be consumed in moderation, they are important for certain physiological functions. These fats are necessary for the production of hormones like progesterone and estrogen, both of which play critical roles in maintaining a healthy pregnancy.

Monounsaturated Fats: These fats, found in foods like avocados, olives, and nuts, provide a good source of energy and contribute to overall heart health. They may be included in a healthy pregnant diet.

Polyunsaturated Fats: Omega-3 and omega-6 fatty acids are crucial for fetal brain development, particularly DHA which is abundant in fatty fish like salmon. Omega-6 fatty acids are also necessary but should be balanced with omega-3s for optimal health.

IV. Dietary Sources of Healthy Fats:

Avocados: A rich source of monounsaturated fats, avocados also provide fiber, folate, and various vitamins and minerals.

Fatty Fish: Excellent sources of omega-3 fatty acids include trout, salmon, mackerel, and sardines. They are essential for the development of the fetal brain.

Nuts and Seeds: Healthy fats, fiber, and vital elements are abundant in almonds, walnuts, chia seeds, and flaxseeds. These can be easily incorporated into a balanced diet.

Olive Oil: Extra virgin olive oil is a healthy source of monounsaturated fats and can be used in cooking or as a dressing.

V. Moderation and Balance:

It is essential to emphasize that while fats are vital, a balanced approach is crucial. Overconsumption of unhealthy fats, such as trans fats and excessive saturated fats from processed foods, should be avoided.

In conclusion, fats play a crucial role in a healthy pregnancy. By incorporating a variety of healthy fats into a balanced diet, pregnant women can support their own health and contribute to the optimal development of their growing foetus.

Remember to consult with a healthcare provider or a registered dietitian for personalized dietary advice during pregnancy. This note is intended for informational purposes only and does not replace professional medical advice.

MICRONUTRIENTS

VITAMINS:

Pregnancy is a transformative phase in a woman's life, marked by numerous physiological changes and an increased demand for essential nutrients. Among these, vitamins play a crucial role in ensuring the health and well-being of both the mother and the developing foetus. These micronutrients are essential for various biological processes, including cell division, tissue formation, and immune function. This article explores the significance of vitamins as micronutrients during pregnancy and highlights their specific roles and sources.

I. Vitamin A:

Vitamin A is essential for vision, immune function, and skin health. During pregnancy, it plays a vital role in the development of the foetal eyes, immune system, and various organs. However, excessive intake of vitamin A can lead to toxicity, so it's crucial to obtain it from natural sources like sweet potatoes, carrots, and leafy greens.

II. Vitamin B-Complex:

Folate (Vitamin B9):

Folate is crucial for preventing neural tube defects in the early stages of fetal development.

Green leafy vegetables, legumes, and fortified grains are excellent sources.

Vitamin B6:

Essential for brain development and function.

Found in meat, fish, whole grains, and bananas.

Vitamin B12: Vital for the formation of red blood cells and neurological development.

mostly found in meat, fish, and dairy products that come from animals.

III. Vitamin C: Vitamin C is an antioxidant that supports tissue repair, collagen production, and iron absorption. It aids in the development of bones and teeth in the foetus. Strawberries, bell peppers, and citrus fruits are all excellent sources of vitamin C.

IV. Vitamin D: Excellent sources of vitamin C are citrus fruits, bell peppers, and strawberries. Inadequate levels can lead to complications such as gestational diabetes and preeclampsia. Natural sources include fatty fish, fortified dairy, and sun exposure.

V. Vitamin E: An antioxidant, vitamin E, protects cells from damage and supports immune function. It is abundant in nuts, seeds, and spinach, among other foods.

VI. Vitamin K: Blood coagulation and bone metabolism require vitamin K. It also supports the development of the foetal circulatory system. Broccoli, Brussels sprouts, and leafy greens are all excellent sources of vitamin K.

VII. Vitamin Biotin: Biotin, a B-vitamin, aids in metabolism and skin health. It's found in eggs, nuts, and certain vegetables.

VIII. Choline: Although not strictly a vitamin, choline is essential for brain development and overall health. Eggs, liver, and peanuts are excellent sources.

Vitamins are indispensable micronutrients that play a pivotal role in pregnancy. Ensuring an adequate intake of these essential nutrients through a balanced diet or, when necessary, through supplements, can significantly contribute to the health and well-being of both the mother and the developing foetus. However, it's crucial to consult a healthcare provider for personalized recommendations to meet individual nutritional needs during pregnancy. By prioritizing a nutrient-rich diet, mothers can provide their infants with the best possible start in life.

MINERALS

Pregnancy is a critical period in a woman's life that demands special attention to nutrition. Adequate intake of essential nutrients, including minerals, is crucial for both the mother's health and the optimal development of the foetus. Minerals, though required in smaller quantities compared to macronutrients like carbohydrates, proteins, and fats, play indispensable roles in various physiological processes. In this comprehensive guide, we will delve into the significance of minerals as micronutrients during pregnancy.

I. Calcium (Ca):

Calcium is vital for the formation and maintenance of strong bones and teeth for both the mother and the developing foetus. It also aids in muscle function, blood clotting, and nerve signaling. A deficiency in calcium during pregnancy can lead to complications like preeclampsia and low birth weight. Good dietary sources include dairy products, fortified plant-based milks, green leafy vegetables, and almonds.

II. Iron (Fe):

Haemoglobin, the protein in charge of carrying oxygen in the blood, is largely composed of iron. During pregnancy, the mother's blood volume increases, necessitating higher iron intake. Iron deficiency anemia can lead to fatigue, weakness, and complications like preterm birth and low birth weight. Foods rich in iron include lean meats, beans, lentils, fortified cereals, and spinach.

III. Zinc (Zn):

Zinc is crucial for DNA synthesis, immune function, and proper growth. It is particularly important in the early stages of pregnancy for cell division and development of organs. Zinc deficiency may lead to impaired fetal growth and an increased risk of preterm delivery. Good dietary sources of zinc include meat, dairy products, whole grains, and legumes.

IV. Magnesium (Mg):

Magnesium is involved in over 300 biochemical reactions in the body, including muscle and nerve function, blood glucose control, and bone health. During pregnancy, magnesium supports the development of the fetal nervous system. Inadequate magnesium intake may contribute to complications like

gestational diabetes and preeclampsia.
Whole grains, nuts, seeds, and leafy green
vegetables are excellent sources of
magnesium.

V. Copper (Cu):

Copper is essential for the formation of
collagen, a structural protein that supports
the development of bones, skin, and
connective tissues. It also plays a role in the
production of red blood cells. A deficiency
in copper during pregnancy can lead to
skeletal abnormalities in the foetus. Foods
rich in copper include shellfish, organ meats,
nuts, and seeds.

VI. Iodine (I):

Iodine is critical for the production of
thyroid hormones, which are essential for
normal brain development and metabolism.
Severe iodine deficiency during pregnancy
can result in intellectual disabilities and
developmental delays in the child. Good
dietary sources include iodized salt, seafood,
dairy products, and eggs.

VII. Selenium (Se):

An essential antioxidant that guards against cell damage is selenium. It also supports the immune system and thyroid function. Adequate selenium intake during pregnancy is associated with a reduced risk of preterm birth and low birth weight. Selenium-rich foods include seafood, lean meats, whole grains, and nuts.

A well-balanced diet rich in a variety of minerals is crucial for a healthy pregnancy. While a diverse and nutrient-dense diet is the best way to obtain these micronutrients, sometimes supplementation may be recommended by healthcare providers, especially if there are specific deficiencies. Consulting a healthcare professional for personalized advice is always recommended. By prioritizing mineral-rich foods, mothers can optimize their own health and support the healthy development of their precious little one.

HYDRATION AND ITS VITAL ROLE IN HEALTHY PREGNANCY

Pregnancy is a transformative and crucial period in a woman's life, marked by a multitude of physiological changes to support the growing fetus. Among the many factors that contribute to a healthy pregnancy, proper hydration stands as one of the cornerstones. This often underestimated aspect plays a pivotal role in ensuring maternal well-being, fetal development, and the overall success of pregnancy.

Physiology of Pregnancy and Increased Fluid Needs

During pregnancy, a woman's body undergoes significant changes to accommodate the developing foetus. Blood volume increases, the heart pumps more blood per minute, and there is a greater demand for nutrients and oxygen. These changes necessitate an expansion of the circulatory system, leading to an increased demand for fluids. Moreover, amniotic fluid, which surrounds and protects the fetus, is primarily composed of water. This reinforces the importance of maintaining optimal hydration levels.

Benefits of Adequate Hydration in Pregnancy

1. Foetal Development: Adequate hydration facilitates the transportation of essential nutrients to the foetus. It helps in the formation of the placenta, which is responsible for supplying oxygen and nutrients to the developing baby. Additionally, amniotic fluid, which acts as a cushion for the fetus, depends heavily on maternal hydration.

2. Prevention of Birth Defects: Studies have shown a correlation between dehydration during pregnancy and an increased risk of neural tube defects, such as spina bifida. Ensuring proper hydration can significantly reduce this risk.

3. Prevention of Preterm Labor: Dehydration may lead to uterine contractions, potentially triggering preterm labour. Maintaining optimal fluid intake can help prevent this, contributing to a full-term pregnancy.

4. Reduction of Urinary Tract Infections (UTIs):

Pregnant women are more susceptible to UTIs due to hormonal changes that affect the urinary tract. Adequate hydration helps to dilute urine, reducing the risk of bacterial growth and subsequent infections.

5. Circulatory Support:

Proper hydration aids in maintaining healthy blood pressure levels, which is crucial for both maternal and foetal well-being. It also supports the expanded blood volume needed during pregnancy.

6. Prevention of Constipation and Hemorrhoids:

Constipation is a common concern in pregnancy, exacerbated by hormonal changes. Sufficient fluid intake helps soften stools and prevent constipation. Thus, there is a lower chance of hemorrhoids forming.

Practical Tips for Maintaining Hydration in Pregnancy

Monitor Urine Color: Pale or straw-colored urine is a good indicator of adequate hydration. Darker urine may signal a need for increased fluid intake.

Frequent Small Sips: Aim to sip water throughout the day rather than consuming large quantities at once. This ensures a steady intake.

Incorporate Hydrating Foods: Fruits and vegetables with high water content (e.g., watermelon, cucumbers) are excellent sources of hydration.

Limit Caffeine: Excessive caffeine can lead to dehydration. Instead, choose decaffeinated beverages and herbal teas.

Avoid Sugary Drinks: These can lead to spikes and crashes in blood sugar levels, potentially causing discomfort and dehydration.

Listen to Your Body: Thirst is a clear signal that your body needs more fluids. Pay close attention to these cues and act quickly.

Account for Physical Activity: If engaged in regular exercise, increase fluid intake to compensate for additional fluid loss through sweating.

Consult Your Healthcare Provider: Individual fluid needs may vary based on factors like activity level, climate, and underlying health conditions. Your healthcare practitioner might make recommendations that are specific to you.

In conclusion, proper hydration is a fundamental aspect of a healthy pregnancy. It supports maternal health, fetal development, and the overall success of the pregnancy journey. By being mindful of fluid intake and making conscious efforts to stay hydrated, expecting mothers can contribute significantly to their own well-being and that of their growing baby. Remember, a well-hydrated pregnancy is a healthy pregnancy.

CONCLUSION

As we reach the conclusion of this journey through "Real Food for Pregnancy," I am filled with gratitude that you've chosen to embark on this transformative path towards a healthier, more vibrant pregnancy. Together, we've explored the profound impact that nourishing, whole foods can have on the well-being of both you and your growing baby. We've delved into the science behind optimal nutrition during this crucial time, and we've unearthed practical strategies to implement these principles into your everyday life.

Throughout this book, I've strived to empower you with knowledge, dispelling myths and providing evidence-based insights into the intricate dance between nutrition and pregnancy. We've celebrated the remarkable potential of nutrient-dense foods, the vital importance of balance, and the significance of mindful eating practices. Together, we've shattered the notion that healthy eating during pregnancy must be burdensome or restrictive, and instead, we've discovered a vibrant and delicious world of nourishment.

Remember, this journey is not about perfection, but about progress. It's about making conscious choices that align with your body's unique needs and respecting the incredible wisdom it holds. By tuning into your own intuition and listening closely to what your body craves, you're setting the stage for a pregnancy filled with vitality and vitality that will resonate long after your little one arrives.

As you move forward, I encourage you to trust in the innate wisdom of your body. Let it be your guide, and let the nourishing foods on your plate be your allies in this extraordinary journey. Embrace each meal as an opportunity to provide your baby with the best possible start in life and to cultivate a foundation of health that will carry them through the years ahead.

I am deeply honored to have been a part of your pregnancy journey, and I have every confidence that you are now equipped with the knowledge and tools to make informed, nourishing choices for yourself and your growing family. May this book serve as a trusted companion, a source of inspiration, and a reminder that you possess the power to create a legacy of health and wellness for generations to come.

With heartfelt wishes for a pregnancy filled with joy, vitality, and abundance.